Essential Oils
50 Summer Diffuser Recipes and Blends

Table of content

Introduction

If you've read my first blog on suggestions for green cleaning with essential oils, you know I strongly discourage the use of chemical cleansers and pesticides. But living with colonies of unwanted critters isn't exactly how I like to spend my summers. As with all my green cleaning solutions, I use the natural insecticidal powers of essential oils.

During the spring and summer months, diffuse 3 drops each of Youthful Living Lavender, Lemon and Peppermint Essential Oils to help support normal respiration and a healthy immune function.

To help purify the air in your home, try diffusing 6 drops of Young Living Purification Combination.

Summer smells can often be overpowering. They're either sickly sweet and fruity or cloyingly floral. By making your own diffuser you can take control of your house's aroma.

You can make this with any empty bottles around your house. We found this adorable small milk bottle that was previously used as a vase. Olive Oil bottles also work perfectly. Reed sticks are easy to find in any craft store, but you can also use bamboo skewers from your grocery store.

Summer! It's that time of year to relax out on the veranda, sip some lavender iced tea, and watch the sun slowly dip behind the tree line.

If you've read my first blog on suggestions for green cleaning with essential oils, you know I strongly discourage the use of chemical cleansers and pesticides. But living with colonies of unwanted critters isn't exactly how I like to spend my summers. As with all my green cleaning solutions, I use the natural insecticidal powers of essential oils.

Chapter 1 – Summer Diffuser Recipes and Blends 1 to 10

1. Citrus Odor for Any room

Lemon – 10 drops

Tangerine – 4 drops

Mandarin – 3 drops

Patchouli – 3 drops

Mix all in an amber bottle, then use in any room diffuser of your choice. Tealight diffusers or electric warmers are ideal for this particular room odor.

2. Jitters Combine

For Jitters when attending summer weddings, parties or other gatherings where strangers could be present – this combination gives you courage to begin conversations! Set in a Personal inhaler or use on a tissue.

Spearmint – 5 drops

Basil – 2 drops

Mix all in an glass bottle, then add to your Personal inhaler.

3. RELIEF for Tired Feet and lower Legs

Being on your feet at play or at work is able to make your feet and ankles quite tired. By soaking in a tepid foot bath where you've added several drops of this blend give them a little relief.

This recipe makes enough for 2-3 foot soaks as you simply need to add 3-4 drops in your foot soak bowl. Add a little Epsom or bath salts to the bowl too.

Spruce needle – 3 drops

Tea Tree – 2 drops

Mix all in an amber bottle. Add 2-4 drops to your own foot soak basin. Relax and enjoy!

4. Remove Odors in a Musty Basement Spray or Diffuser Incorporation

Lime – 10 drops

Lavender – 10 drops

Cedarwood – 10 drops

Coconut Emulsifier - 2 1/2 teaspoonsful

Combine the above in a amber bottle subsequently mix 50 drops with ½ teaspoon coconut emulsifier. Pour into your PET plastic spray bottle and add 4 oz of water. Shake well and spray onto any surface in your cellar that seems to be growing the unwanted odor. Spray some around the area also. As a substitute it is possible to utilize this incorporation in a diffuser (omit the emulsifier as well as the water) - such as a SpaScenter or Tru Melange and diffuser continuously for many days.

5. CLOTHING IN the Cedar Cabinet Odor

Cedarwood Atlas – 40 drops

Clove bud – 15 drops

Orange – 15 drops

Blend these in an amber bottle. Afterward put several drops on a Terra Cotta Disc diffuser and allow it to soak in. Then simply place in the corner or on a shelf in your cabinet.

This really is an odor that is great, in case you enjoy the scent of Cedarwood.

6. For a fast summer Hot Tub or Bath Combine

Vanilla in Jojoba – 10 drops
Lavender – 4 drops
Juniper berry – 2 drops
Blend together in an amber bottle. Then add the entire contents to your tub. If you use this combination in a very large bathtub, you'll should double this recipe for a 4 person bath.

7. STINKY Carpeting Refresher

High humidity and all the bacteria and mold that could lurk in your carpeting can soon make the room smell badly. Blend this up and use before vacuuming to freshen not just the atmosphere but your carpet!

Lime – 1 teaspoonful (5ml)
Tangerine – ½ teaspoonful (2 1/2 ml)
Litsea Cubeba – ¼ teaspoonful (1 1/4 ml)
Mix all the ingredients together in a Glass pint jar. Shake well, let mixture for 24 hours. Then sprinkle on your own carpet, let sit for 20-30 minutes. Vacuum your carpet as usual.

Keep any remaining scented powder in a tightly covered jar in the refrigerator. You might need to make fresh or even used within 2-3 weeks.

8. Amazing Summer Body Spray

Vanilla Absolute Pure – 4 drops

The S'WOODS – 10 drops

Litsea Cubeba – 5 drops

Coconut Emulsifier – 30 drops

Body spray unscented Base – 2 ounces

Empty PET plastic bottle

In a 2 oz PET bottle, combine the essential oils and add the emulsifier to this. Then add 2 ounces of our unscented body spray. Shake well.

Spray in your body after bathing or showering, or some time you feel you would like to freshen up your scent!

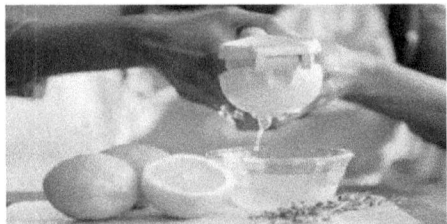

9. Seasonal Support Fusion

Attempt this during spring as well as summer for helping maintain clear breathing and a healthy immune response.

2 drops lavender essential oil

2 drops lemon essential oil

2 drops peppermint essential oil

10.   Citrus Explosion Blend

Diffusing citrus combines consistently makes the home odor happy and clean.

1 drop lemon essential oil

2 drops wild orange essential oil

1 drop lime essential oil

Chapter 2 – Summer Diffuser Recipes and Blends 11 to 20

11. Fresh and Clean Mix

Create a welcoming feeling in your home with this one:
2 drops lavender essential oil
2 drops lemon essential oil
2 drops rosemary essential oil

12. Scent Eliminator Fusion

Great for removing any smells in the house
2 drops lemon essential oil
2 drops melaleuca essential oil
1 drop cilantro essential oil
1 drop lime essential oil

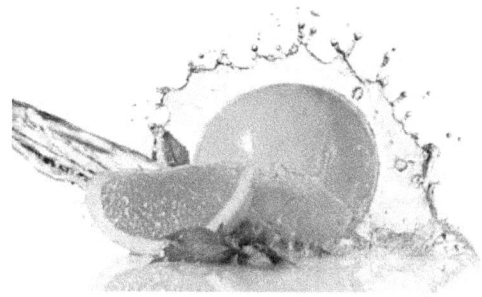

13. Flower Garden Essential Oil Diffuser Recipe

Makes your house smell like a flower garden
1 drop geranium essential oil

2 drops lavender essential oil

2 drops roman chamomile essential oil

14. Let's Focus Blend

Perfect for increasing alertness, or when you'll need a fast pick-me-up:

2 drops wild orange essential oil

2 drops peppermint essential oil

15. Get Focused

Diffuse to get your head in the game.

2 drops Peppermint

2 drops Cinnamon

1 drop Rosemary

16. Calming Diffusing Fusion

Helps everyone calm down and relax

3 drops Lavender

3 drops Geranium

2 drops Clary Sage

2 drops Ylang Ylang

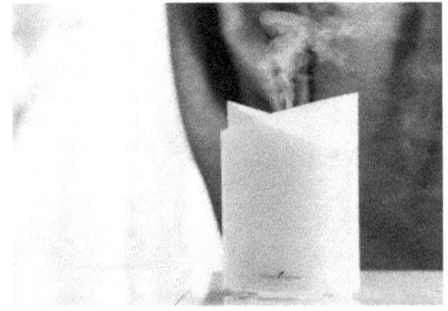

17. Headache Relief

Diffuse to help relieve a terrible headache
1-2 drops Marjoram
1-2 drops Thyme
1-2 drops Rosemary
1-2 drops Peppermint
1-2 drops Lavender

18. Grounding Essential Oil Diffuser Recipe

If you're planning to relax nicely
2 drops essential oil vetiver
2 drops essential oil cedar wood

19. Holiday Bliss

Get ready for the Holidays with this delightful mix!
2 drops Cassia
2 drops Wild Orange

20.   Winter Woods Combine

Will remind you of a walk through the woods. It's perfect for the holidays!
2 drops cedar wood
2 drops white fir
2 drops cypress
2 drops wintergreen

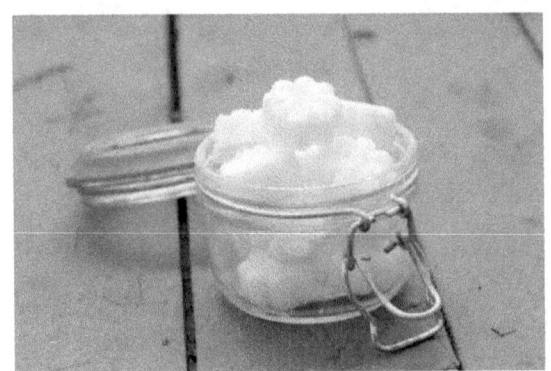

Chapter 3 – Summer Diffuser Recipes and Blends 21 to 30

21. Spiced Cider

Even when it's not drop, this really is a fantastic one to use to relax and ground you.

4 drops Wild Orange

3 drops Cinnamon

3 drops Ginger

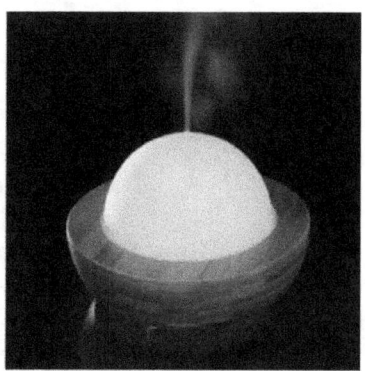

22.   Sick of Being Sick Blend

When you are feeling under the weather, try this germ fighting and mood boosting blend!

2 drops OnGuard Blend

2 drops frankincense

2 drops lemon

23.   Immune Booster

A perfect option during cold and flu season:

1 drop rosemary essential oil

1 drop clove essential oil

1 drop eucalyptus essential oil

1 drop cinnamon bark essential oil

1 drop wild orange essential oil

24.   Emotional Healing Blend

Just what you need to soothe the emotions.

2 drops Wild Orange

2 drops Bergamot

2 drops Cypress

2 drops Frankincense

Get Happy Blend

It's pure happiness.

2 drops lemon

2 drops wild orange

2 drops bergamot

2 drops grapefruit

25.   Be Happy

A great mood-boosting blend.

3 drops Bergamot

2 drops Geranium

3 drops Lavender

26.   Wake Up Productive

Stimulating and helps increases mental alertness.

4 drops Wild Orange
4 drops Peppermint

27.   Sunshine Bliss

A little burst of sunshine.
3 drops Wild Orange
3 drops Grapefruit
2 drops Lemon
1 drop Bergamot

28.   The Energizer

Diffuse this one first thing in the morning for a big boost:
2 drops wild orange essential oil
2 drops frankincense essential oil
2 drops cinnamon essential oil

29.   Forest Air Freshening Blend

Blend together:
Spruce - 50 drops
Lavender - 25 drops
Cedarwood - 20 drops
Add combination to diffuser and diffuse for a woods fresh scent!

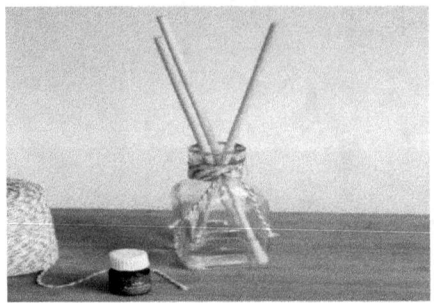

30.   Romantic Mix

Mix together:

Palmarosa - 24 drops

Ylang ylang - 3 drops

Clary sage - 6 drops

Nutmeg - 6 drops

Lime - 12 drops

Add mixture to diffuser and diffuse.

Chapter 4 – Summer Diffuser Recipes and Blends 31 to 40

31. Heavy Relaxation Blend

Combine together:
Lavender - 30 drops
Marjoram - 10 drops
Mandarin - 5 drops
Add blend to diffuser and diffuse for actual relaxation!

32. Diffuser Mountain Blend

We're attracted to this mix because we're starting the month of August in the beautiful mountains of the High Sierras that encompass Lake Tahoe.

33. Lake Diffuser Blend

We spent the day at the lake, paddle boarding and swimming. When we got home, this blend went in the diffuser to continue our experience of outdoor enjoyment and time in sunlight. Use it whenever you need a pick me up or when the weather isn't amazing to bring summer indoors.

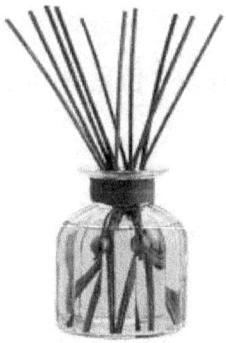

34.   Burnout Buster Combination

Try this blend when you've been working hard and want only a little self-care and equilibrium. When it's just been one of those days. When you need to find some energy, to get rejuvenated, and to keep going another day. Vetiver is excellent for centering and grounding. Lavender is calming and relaxing. And Bergamot supports self-acceptance and confidence. This will be a goto combine for all of us who desire just a little help sometimes. And some time at the shore doesn't hurt either.

35.   Italian Summer Blend

Italian Summer. This is probably my very favorite blend of essential oils for the diffuser. Lemon is great for focus and mood boosting, Cypress supports movement and stream, and Bergamot is refreshing and can help to alleviate pressure and anxiety. Odors like a hot tub, it's so celestial.

36.   Snooze Mix

One of many slumber blends for a restful night. This one is delightful and perfect for children and grownups equally. This is my daughter's go to oil for nighttime, and Sandalwood – great for yoga, meditation, and settling the mind.

37.   Experience Portmanteau

Today found us cruising a water taxi across an alpine lake and hiking with our kids on one of the most famous trails in the world – the Pacific Crest Trail. We were up for experience after diffusing this invigorating experience blend! Plan an outside trip and seize the day!

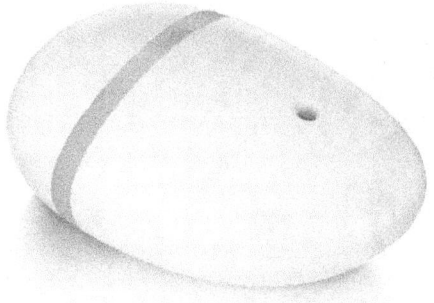

38.   Don't Trouble Me Mix

The Don't Trouble Me Mixture... Crucial for those times when you need some alone time. At our houses, we have a "don't trouble me" chair, which is not to say others aren't welcome...or perhaps they aren't, merely for small touch. Curl up with this combination and an excellent book and settle into yourself. Just you. Only for a little while. They'll comprehend.

39.   Release Mix

Need to release something or detox head or body? This week, we did three things to support release. First, we used the mantra of "launch" during meditation practice to let go of narratives that come up. Second, we practiced "tremoring" as a way to release tension in the psoas (fight or flight) muscle...very interesting items.

40.   Clean House Mix

Only cleaned the house? Or even only one corner? Add this to the end of your clean routine as a benefit and final touch for your attempts. Completely sweet and pleasing.

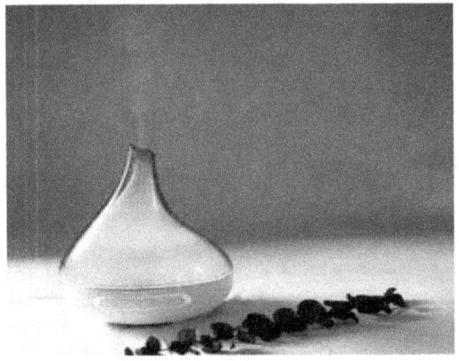

Chapter 5 – Summer Diffuser Recipes and Blends 41 to 50

41. Worry Less Mix

This could be used as an "fury control" mix to bring things back into perspective. Bergamot for hope and cleanse, Rosemary for assurance during times of great change, White Fir for busting negative patterns of behavior, and Peppermint for a "breather" when a reprieve from emotional tough times is needed.

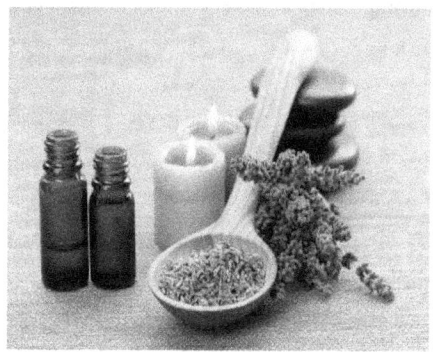

42.   Up and At 'Em Blend

I was up and on my mat early this morning, and used this focus and energy blend of an Invigorating Citrus mix and peppermint for some pep. All BEFORE a screen gets turned on. Try it and see how your outlook and productivity changes.

43.   Beat the Heat Combination

It was a scorcher here in the Bay Area!! This combo which is classic has 2 essential oils heavy hitter, Lavender and Peppermint help cool the body down and are wonderful in a diffuser. Tomorrow is goanna be a hot one too...stay cool

44.   Stay Healthy Fusion

When everyone heads back to school, it's even more important to support the body consequently no school days are missed!!! Keep your immune system strong and healthy with this simple diffuser combination using this Resistance Blend and Wild Orange. The Immunity Combination comprises Wild Orange Peel, Clove Bud, Cinnamon Bark, Eucalyptus, and Rosemary, and supports a healthy immune function. The inclusion of Wild Orange uplifts the mind and body, as well as acting as a strong cleanser and purifying agent. Collectively, this blend protects against seasonal and environmental hazards and is full of antioxidants to keep you and yours going strong. This is day-to-day oil in our house.

45.   Assignments Fusion

Lots of kiddos going back to school!
Lemon – the oil of focus, nourishes the head and help attention
Basil – assists with overwhelm and exhaustion, and rejuvenates after burnout
Rosemary – the oil of knowledge and transition, supports the assimilation of new information & encounters
Cypress – helps those who are psychologically or emotionally stuck, or with perfectionistic tendencies to let things unfold naturally
Peppermint – fosters the mood in times of discouragement, and invigorates the body, mind, and spirit.

46.   TGIF Combination

Geranium – directs us away from the rational mind and into the warmth and nurture of the heart

Lemongrass – cleanses the energy within a room or space so we can move forward

Cypress – the oil of movement and flow, helps us cast aside stresses and let go of control

Grapefruit – Supports us to honor our physical needs (a glass of wine, anyone?? But just enough!!)

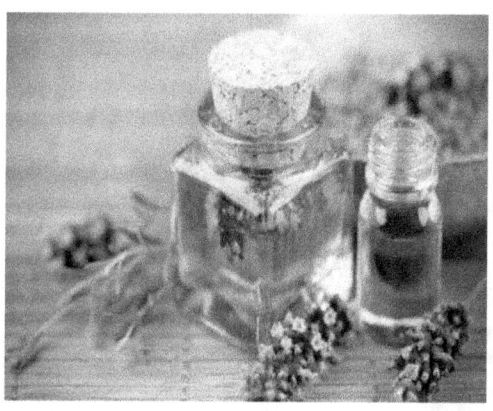

47.   Flowery Rush

Attempt this delightful and uplifting flowery odor.

20 drops Jasmine

15 drops Royal Hawaiian™ Sandalwood

6 drops Frankincense

3 drops Idaho Balsam Fir

48.   Solstice Radiance

Clary Sage - Youthful Living

8 drops Blue Cypress

5 drops Bergamot

5 drops Cedar wood

1 drop Clary Sage

49.   Citrus Summer

Invigorate and refresh your spirit with this sunny aroma.

Palo Santo - Youthful Living10 drops Hinoki

8 drops Myrrh

5 drops Citrus Fresh™

1 drop Juniper

1 drop Vetiver

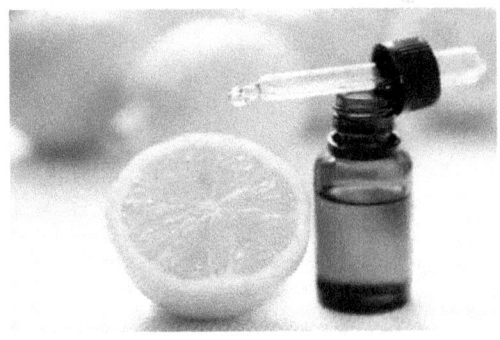

50.   Sunny Bouquet

Ylang Ylang - Youthful Living Freshen any space with this cornucopia of smells.

1 drop Ravintsara

1 drop Eucalyptus Globulus

Chapter 6 – What Essential Oils Can Do For You

Essential oils are chemical compounds with aromatic properties found in the seeds, roots, stalks, bark, blossoms, and other parts of plants. For centuries, there are many narratives of healing properties of these precious oils. There were also many means essential oils were extracted out of distinct plants. As an example, rose oil was expressed by massaging leaves with animal fat. The vast majority of oils from plants are steam distilled at a certain temperature and a particular pressure. The most healing oils with optimum advantages are taken after the first distillation. I don't recommend purchasing any oils from any other distillation. Some companies will do additional distillation to enhance the oil's scent, but the chemical compounds of the plant have been changed. YIKES! A lot of companies also create independent testing reports on the oils and even security reports. Comprehend there isn't any regulation in purity or potency of essential oils, so these resources are amazingly valuable.

How can you use essential oils after you find a fantastic company?
Aromatic use is very safe. Always make sure that the diffuser you purchase is compatible with the oils you purchase. Cleaning the diffuser with each kind of oil you use might also be in order, but many companies have improved on the diffusers used and cleaning is not required every time you change oils. Aromatic use is a terrific way to freshen halls, lavatories, and other areas. I love diffusing oils when company is over or in my bedroom to help out with rest.

Topical use is, in addition, quite common and safe. The only contentious topic of topical use is neat application. Awesome application happens when the essential oils are put directly on the skin without dilution. Many companies say that most of their oils are safe for fantastic program. Essential oils are QUITE strong. An individual drop of oil is equal to seventy-five cups of tea with that particular plants. Such potency can be a problem with skin discomfort. The most significant rule with essential oils is always to dilute in carrier oils. Carrier oils are plant based fatty oils used to dilute essential oils. A great rule of thumb would be to always perform a skin patch test using 1 drop essential oil and 1ml carrier oil.

Thus, if you've 5ml carrier oil (or 1 teaspoon), 5 drops of essential oil is the maximum to maintain the 5% solution. There are many safe carrier oils like vegetable oil, coconut oil, sweet almond oil, grape seed oil, jojoba oil, olive oil, and other oils. If you have a vitamin E allergy, Jojoba oil is a fantastic option. If you or a family member has an allergy to nuts, please check for nut based oils in fusion and steer clear of almond and coconut carrier oils. Ingredients should be recorded on labels; nevertheless, it is always a safe idea to call the companies directly. Use extra caution with youthful skin, aged skin, sensitive skin, damaged skin, inflamed skin, and especially diseased skin. These skin types absorb more oil and are usually sensitive to the potency. People who have sensitive skin should avoid external use of Wintergreen, peppermint, and birch. Aromatic uses are safe for pregnant girls, but care should be revealed with external application, particularly in the first three months. Pregnant women should avoid the following oils: Aniseed, Basil, Birth, Camphor, Hyssop, Mugwort, Parsley seed or leaf, Pennroyal, Sage, Tansy, Tarragon, Wintergreen, Wormwood, Thuja, Clary Sage, and any other oil with phytoestrogen qualities. Internal use is also not recommended for pregnant girls. If reaction occurs, dilute with carrier oils, not water. No essential oils on children younger than 18 months. Always keep oils out of reach of children.

Some publications suggest topical application on pets. Do not use essential oils on pets. They cannot handle the potency. Some oils that are totally safe for us have been revealed to be highly toxic for animals. Oils including terpenes, like lavender an thyme, can cause liver and/or kidney failure in cats. Lavender and Thyme have been lauded in some novels as wonderful flea and tick control. Tansy has been poisonous to both cattle and horses. Use caution around pets. Accidental exposure may happen, observe your pet for any signs of distress. Some of my creatures have licked where I 've set oils on my feet, and they had no problems at all.

Internal use is the most controversial topic of aromatherapy. A lot of reputable companies support internal use, nevertheless, most Aromatherapy and Herbal Associations, for instance, International Federation of Aromatherapists (IFA) contraindicate internal use of essential oils within their code of ethics by health care providers. The National Association of Holistic Aromatherapy discourages Aromatherapists of using essential oils internally unless trained to do that. They are currently exploring the security of internal use.

Essential Oils are the essence of the plant and are never derived from an animal source. This doesn't mean that I advocate vegetarianism or veganism as that is a specific choice with it's own dietary needs and options. Nevertheless, essential oils are a good means for vegetarians and vegans to supplement what they may be lacking within their diets unless they grow all their food themselves, but I digress. Essential oils are part of the Alternative Medicine class but are becoming more and more relevant in Traditional Medicine as scientists are realizing the value of these very fundamental materials because of their wide assortment of components.

Essential oils are natural aromatic compounds found in the various parts of the plant, from the bark to the roots to the leaves to the flowers. They can be both beautifully and powerfully fragrant. If you've ever appreciated the gift of a rose, walked by a field of lavender or the fresh smell of cut mint then you've experienced the aromatic qualities of essential oils. Essential oils are ten times more powerful and wholesome than their dehydrated herbal counterparts that are often bottled and scattered to give food unique flavors and scents. These fundamental oils give the plants they are found in a distinctive odor but also provide protection against predators and help in pollination.

Essential oils are non water-based phytochemicals made up of volatile organic compounds. Although they are fat soluble, they do not contain oily lipids or acids found in vegetable and animal oils. If they're in their pure form, they will never make an oily deposit or sensation on the skin.

In addition to their intrinsic advantages to plants and being delightfully fragrant to folks, essential oils are used throughout history in many cultures for their medicinal and healing benefits. Modern scientific study and trends towards more holistic approaches to wellness are driving a revival and new discovery of essential oil wellbeing applications. The Egyptians were some of the first individuals to use aromatic essential oils widely in medical practice, beauty treatment, food preparation, and in religious ceremony.

Getting colds is extremely uncomfortable and annoying. The cold causes nasal drainage, down and coughing time. Preventing a cold is the easiest means to cope with a cold but what do you do if you get a cold. Using Eucalyptus essential oils are able to help you overcome a cold. I know they have helped me.

Occasionally, I've gotten a summer cold being with a cold around a friend. Sadly not expecting to get a cold at that time of year I was not prepared. When it did occur I promptly used the oils and the cold passed instantly. I know which oils carried even though that has not occurred in an extended time. As long as I use the essential oils I don't get colds.

Preventing colds needs investment of time and effort when you do not have to experience making a physician visit, coughing, and blowing your nose but it pays off. Using the different Eucalyptus essential oils can help you protect against catching a cold and build protection.

The pleasant aromas of summer comprise the aromatic aroma of honey suckle and the fragrant purple blooms of lavender floating in the warm breeze and the moist summer aroma rising from the freshly cut yard, the clean scent of the just washed towels drying in the sun and the fresh ocean breeze wafting coconut and citrus. Usually, the summer aromas take you.

Fragrance is a strong way of immediately changing our mood. Life usually abounds during summer the air is full of aromatic fragrances and as the flowers, trees and the herbs are in full bloom. But when this same summer that is aromatic turns warm and muggy afterward most of our houses can use a small summer smell to feel fresh. Clean summer scents can do a lot to us, but it's very harmful to rely on the Plugin air fresheners as well as the sprays, as both contain harmful chemicals, which can cause damage if inhaled. Instead we should rely on the wisdom of our great grandmothers and use natural products to make our homes smell refreshing and clean.

Hence let the delightful aroma of the summer melt away your stress and revive body and your mind. Isn't it much better to use essential oils rather than the perfumes made with chemicals? Real essential oils are therapeutic and even have a fuller and yet a lighter caress, as compared to the commercial perfumes.

Zesty Lemon- This lemony clean scent lifts your spirits up and can boost. So try rubbing against it or even you are able to attempt wrenching the peel to release the scent into the room and only peeling lemon. You can even distribute the lemony fragrance by simmering the lemon slices in the water on the stove.

Place dried lavender in an attractive container and place it next to your bed, to make your bedroom smell fresh and warm. This scent promotes sound sleep with dreams that are peaceful.

Rosemary Blotch- Attempt burning some sprigs of dried rosemary using an ashtray and as this smell disperses into the atmosphere in your house it turns refreshing and this technique is used from past many centuries since its anti-microbial, in sickrooms.

Sweet smelling Green Mist- Sprays and Mists are the simplest ways to incorporate aroma that is natural to fight germs and your house. By using essential oils mists and sprays disperse aromatherapy. Nothing could be simpler than spraying on several drops on bathroom surfaces or the doorknobs, telephones. Your sweet home will not smell stale also.

The smell remover, vanilla - The vanilla bean has the properties to reduce scent so try this superb trick to remove unwanted odors out of your house.

Tricky Cinnamon- Attempt filling a pot with ground cinnamon and enjoy the wafts of the sweet scent daylong.

Conclusion

Essential oils are a curiosity to many folks -- they smell fine, but they're simply unsure what to do with them, never mind ways to get the most from aromatherapy's science-established advantages (like antiviral, antibacterial and pressure-reducing activities). So where to start?! Inhale! Breathe them in! We are going to start with a quick review of the possible benefits of diffusing essential oils for your family, with special notes for children, then look at the finest diffusers for each use.

They have proven antibacterial and antiviral actions; they are able to ruin these microbes in the air, while simultaneously support the strength of our immune system. There is a good bit of scientific data backing both these claims available for free viewing at PubMed.Gov -- start by simply searching for "essential oil" and see where it takes you. Again, the simplest way to reap these benefits of essential oils is to use a diffuser to release the oils into the air in your surroundings. A diffuser simply evaporates oils faster than they'd naturally, getting a healing concentration into your living or office space -- but there are many diffuser styles -- we'll help you find the one best suited to your needs.

Diffusers For Antiviral/Antimicrobial Activity & Immune Support

For disinfecting the air in your environment, you have to evaporate a comparatively high concentration of essential oils. The only way to do this effectively, while preserving the oils to keep costs to a minimum is to use a "nebulizing" diffuser in conjunction with a timer system. While these diffusers will have a somewhat higher initial cost, they are the only diffusers that will result "therapeutic" doses of essential oils for every possible use. This is also the diffuser that will diffuse aroma in the biggest area; so even if you just need a pleasing aroma in your house, for over 800 square feet, this is the diffuser of choice.

The nebulizers come in two fashions: "cold air" and "ultrasonic". The cold air units use only air pressure to diffuse the oils, and outcome the greatest concentration of any diffuser sort. The ultrasonic is essentially a small water-humidification unit, where oils are mixed with water and then evaporated. Both fashions generally have output controls, so you can turn up or down the amount of oil being diffused. They are also both extremely quiet.

Diffusers for "Smell"-therapy: Anti-Stress and Mental Support

For easy aromatic use -- where oils are used for uplifting your spirits, relaxing or helping your children sleep, or simply making your environment smell fabulous, a "fan" or "warming" diffuser is absolutely suitable. The fan units will emit a quiet hum when on, the heating units will be hushed -- and the fan units will normally emit aroma into a fairly sized space, while the less-expensive heating units are satisfied for an individual room.

Use Oils Economically with a Timer

The best means to use the least number of essential oil for your needs is to use a timer -- either built in to the diffuser or a readily available appliance timer. Aromatically, your "smell scent" will become fast accustom to the odor, and you will start to believe the diffuser isn't operating anymore. Running the diffuser for only a couple of minutes every half an hour lets your nose "forget" the oils are in the air. The same principal works for disinfecting the atmosphere and immune system support -- there is no need to over-saturate the air with essential oils. They are so potent that there is no need to continuously diffuse a high concentration for these effects.

Selecting Oils For Your Goal

All essential oils have naturally distinct chemical make-ups. That is what gives them their individual odors and their individual healing activities. For an uplifting, pleasing setting, the "evergreen" oils are very fine: Fir Needle, Spruce, and Juniper Berry. These are exceptional antidepressant aromatics also, along with the citrus oils: Bergamot, Orange, Lemon, Grapefruit and the like, plus Rose and other uplifting flower-scents. For quieting and better rest, Lavender is the first choice; when people aren't a fan of this popular floral oil, Sandalwood and Ylang Ylang are excellent alternatives. For all the goals, its crucial that you use oils you or your family really like the odor of! There are MANY oils to choose from, and by sampling a few, you're sure to find something everyone appreciates.

FREE Bonus Reminder

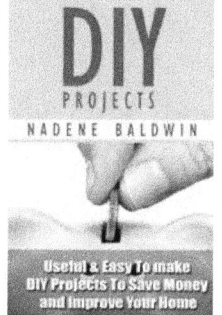

If you have not grabbed it yet, please go ahead and download your special bonus report *"DIY Projects. 13 Useful & Easy To Make DIY Projects To Save Money & Improve Your Home!"*
Simply Click the Button Below

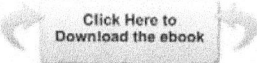

OR **Go to This Page**
http://diyhomecraft.com/free

BONUS #2: More Free & Discounted Books
Do you want to receive more Free & Discounted Books?
We have a mailing list where we send out our new Books when they go free or with a discount on Kindle. Click on the link below to sign up for Free & Discount Book Promotions.
=> Sign Up for Free & Discount Book Promotions <=

OR Go to this URL

http://zbit.ly/1WBb1Ek

www.ingramcontent.com/pod-product-compliance
Lightning Source LLC
Chambersburg PA
CBHW072021290526
45787CB00013B/1661